PFIZER'S EFFICACY ILLUSION

The 0.84% Truth

Alex Exum

Park Dale Press

ISBN: 9798398625103
Imprint: Independently published

Cover design by: Art Painter
Library of Congress Control Number: 2018675309
Printed in the United States of America

FOREWORD

In a world marked by constant noise and distraction, we often find ourselves trusting what is presented to us without delving deeper into the undercurrents that shape the narratives. This book is a product of my journey to unearth the truth beneath the dazzling facade of data and statistics that characterized one of the most pivotal moments in recent history – the advent of Pfizer's COVID-19 vaccine.

The story unfolded like a suspense novel, with a promise of 95% protection that stirred hope across the globe. Yet, as I found, reality was a stark contrast, veiled beneath layers of complex scientific parlance and skewed representations. The task was to unravel this entangled ball of yarn, to seek out the Absolute Risk Reduction that lay obscured in the shadows of its more popular counterpart, the Relative Risk Reduction.

None of this would have been possible without the diligent work of the Canadian Covid Care Alliance. Their unwavering commitment to transparency and truth in public health was the lighthouse that guided my journey through the stormy seas of complex health data. Their work inspired me to dig deeper, to ask the tough questions, and not to accept the surface narrative at face value. For this, I owe them a debt of gratitude. They woke me up to the reality of this deception, empowering me with the tools to navigate the intricate labyrinth of scientific literature.

To my readers, I offer this book as an exploration, a journey into the heart of a complex issue. It's not intended to sow doubt or mistrust, but rather to inspire a culture of inquiry and critical thinking. It's a call to action for each of us to engage with scientific data more critically, to question the narratives presented to us, and to make informed decisions that consider every aspect of the evidence before us.

As you flip through these pages, I encourage you to approach the content with an open mind. Our world is complex, and so too are the issues we grapple with. By shedding light on one such instance of misrepresentation, my hope is that we can strive towards greater transparency, trust, and truth in our collective health journey.

With gratitude,

Alex Exum

"If you want to think clearly, always, always find out how many cases were possible before you believe a statistic."

Archbishop Fulton J. Sheen

CHAPTER 1: THE BIG PROMISE

In a world gripped by the COVID-19 pandemic, hope arrived in the form of a vial. Pfizer's vaccine emerged as the torchbearer in the fight against the coronavirus, an elixir that promised to lead humanity out of the dark tunnel of uncertainty, sickness, and death. Its launch was accompanied by a bold claim that sparked optimism in the hearts of billions around the world - a dazzling 95% efficacy rate.

News of this high efficacy was swiftly disseminated across media channels globally, engendering an atmosphere of triumph. The breakthrough was lauded in international headlines, leading news bulletins, and social media feeds, making it nearly impossible to ignore. Pfizer's vaccine was not just a scientific marvel; it had quickly become a symbol of human resilience and the promise of a return to normalcy.

Government health agencies, scientists, and medical professionals echoed the 95% figure with unequivocal certainty. This unanimous endorsement by the scientific community further bolstered public confidence. The number became a beacon of hope for a beleaguered global populace eager to break free from the virus's stranglehold.

And why wouldn't it? In the face of an unprecedented global

health crisis, the thought of a vaccine with a 95% efficacy rate seemed nothing short of miraculous. It promised an imminent end to the pandemic, the resumption of pre-COVID life, and the safety of our loved ones. This impressive figure, 95%, was more than a statistic; it was the embodiment of hope, security, and freedom.

For the everyday person, understanding the intricacies of vaccine efficacy or the complexity of the pharmaceutical trials was far less critical than the beacon of hope the 95% offered. The widespread acceptance of the Pfizer vaccine was, in part, a testament to the power of that promise. It stood as an undisputed truth, a savior in desperate times.

As Pfizer's vaccine rolled out across the globe, inoculating millions, the collective sigh of relief was palpable. But beneath this facade of triumph, a significant detail lay hidden, waiting to be unearthed: the real efficacy story was not as straightforward as it seemed. The 95% promise, as we would discover, was based on a particular interpretation of the trial data, an interpretation that allowed a more convenient truth to overshadow a less flattering reality. The stage was set for the grand unmasking of what we now know as Pfizer's Efficacy Illusion.

CHAPTER 2: UNDERSTANDING EFFICACY

In the realm of vaccines and pharmaceuticals, 'efficacy' is a term that often gets thrown around, primarily when speaking about the success of a new drug or intervention. To fully grasp the unfolding narrative of Pfizer's efficacy illusion, we must first understand what efficacy truly means in this context and how it is measured.

Simply put, efficacy refers to how well a vaccine or a drug works under ideal, controlled conditions, typically in a clinical trial. It's a measure of the reduction in disease incidence in a vaccinated group compared to an unvaccinated one. However, there are two primary ways this reduction can be interpreted - through Relative Risk Reduction (RRR) and Absolute Risk Reduction (ARR).

RRR is the reduction in risk in the treated group (say, those who receive a vaccine) compared to the control group (those who don't receive the vaccine) in a clinical trial. It's a percentage that represents the relative decrease in risk between these two groups.

For instance, if in a trial, the risk of disease in the untreated group is 10%, and in the treated group, it is 5%, the RRR would be 50%. This is because the risk of disease in the treated group is half that of the untreated group.

However, the RRR doesn't tell the full story. It's a relative measure that compares two groups, but it doesn't consider the overall risk to an individual. This is where ARR comes in.

The ARR, on the other hand, considers the overall risk reduction for an individual, not just the relative decrease between two groups. It's calculated by subtracting the risk of disease in the treated group from the risk in the untreated group.

In the above example, where the risk in the untreated group was 10%, and in the treated group, it was 5%, the ARR would be 5%. This means that for an individual, the vaccine reduces their overall risk of disease by 5%.

The crucial distinction is that RRR provides a relative measure between two groups and can often sound more impressive, while ARR offers a more individual perspective and can seem less dramatic. Both are technically accurate ways to measure efficacy, but their interpretation and presentation can significantly influence public perception.

Armed with this understanding, we are better equipped to dissect Pfizer's original trial report and the grand efficacy illusion that has been orchestrated.

CHAPTER 3: THE ORIGINAL TRIAL REPORT

Pfizer's vaccine's journey to its celebrated status began with a hefty document: the original trial report. Published in the New England Journal of Medicine, the report delineated the results of the comprehensive clinical trials Pfizer had conducted. It was within the intricate details of this report that the seeds of the efficacy illusion were sown.

The trials enlisted a total of 43,548 participants, a substantial number befitting the magnitude of the task at hand. These participants were divided into two groups: the treatment group, which received the Pfizer inoculation, and the control group, which received a saline solution, effectively a placebo.

This division is a standard practice in clinical trials, serving as a comparison point to evaluate the intervention's effectiveness - in this case, the Pfizer vaccine. It allows researchers to observe the differences between those who receive the vaccine and those who do not.

Over a period of two months, the research team closely monitored these two groups to track the incidence of COVID-19. It's important to note that the trials were conducted when the virus was rampant, and exposure risk was relatively high.

As the two months of the trial came to an end, the data was collected, analyzed, and compiled into the trial report. The reported results seemed impressive. The vaccine appeared to perform exceptionally well, with the treatment group showing significantly lower rates of COVID-19 than the control group. The performance was encapsulated in one headline-grabbing figure: 95% efficacy.

However, a careful examination of the report would reveal that the touted 95% figure was not reflective of Absolute Risk Reduction. Instead, it represented the Relative Risk Reduction between the control group and the treatment group. The Absolute Risk Reduction - a more individual-centric measure - was left lurking in the background, a less glamorous figure largely unnoticed in the public discourse around the vaccine's efficacy.

The report, a technical and scientifically dense document, remained largely inaccessible to the general public. Most people had to rely on interpretations and summaries presented by media outlets and health officials - interpretations that focused overwhelmingly on the 95% RRR figure. The stage was set for the Pfizer efficacy illusion to take hold, with the unassuming 0.84% ARR figure waiting silently in the wings.

CHAPTER 4: THE RELATIVE RISK REDUCTION (RRR)

The 95% efficacy claim - the figure that sparked global hope and confidence - was a product of Relative Risk Reduction. The intricacies of RRR, and the way it contributed to the perception of the Pfizer vaccine's effectiveness, necessitates a deeper dive.

As we previously established, RRR is a comparison of the risk of an event between a control group and a treatment group. In the case of Pfizer's trial, it compared the risk of developing COVID-19 between those who received the vaccine and those who didn't.

In the trial, a small fraction of participants contracted COVID-19 in both groups - but crucially, the incidence was lower in the vaccinated group. To calculate the RRR, researchers observed the relative decrease in risk between the two groups. The result was a remarkable 95% - a figure that suggested the risk of developing COVID-19 was 95% lower in the vaccinated group than in the control group.

While the RRR figure is scientifically valid, it's crucial to understand what it does not tell us. It doesn't provide a measure of an individual's overall risk reduction after receiving the vaccine. Rather, it gives a comparative measure, highlighting the difference in risk between two groups.

This feature of RRR can lead to an inflated perception of a vaccine's effectiveness. When we hear "95% efficacy," it's natural to assume that means the vaccine will protect 95 out of every 100 vaccinated people from the disease. But this is a misinterpretation of RRR. It doesn't mean 95 out of 100 vaccinated individuals are protected, but that the vaccinated group as a whole has a 95% lower risk compared to an unvaccinated group.

By basing their headline efficacy figure on RRR, Pfizer was not doing anything scientifically incorrect or unusual. However, this figure's prominent use in public communication without adequate explanation or context led to widespread misinterpretation and inflated expectations of the vaccine's individual protection level.

Unwittingly, the global public had been entranced by a number that, while scientifically accurate, did not tell the full story of individual protection. The curtain was yet to be lifted on the less celebrated yet equally important figure: the Absolute Risk Reduction.

CHAPTER 5: THE ABSOLUTE RISK REDUCTION (ARR)

In the echo chamber of the 95% efficacy claim, a considerably quieter yet profoundly important number sat largely ignored. This figure, the Absolute Risk Reduction (ARR), offers a different, perhaps more sobering perspective on Pfizer's vaccine's effectiveness. Far from the heady heights of 95%, the ARR for Pfizer's vaccine stood at a humble 0.84%.

What does this number tell us? ARR provides a measure of the overall reduction in risk for an individual receiving the intervention - in this case, the Pfizer vaccine. It's calculated by subtracting the risk of disease in the treated group from the risk in the untreated group. Essentially, it tells us how much the vaccine reduces an individual's overall risk of contracting COVID-19.

In the context of Pfizer's trial, let's consider some hypothetical numbers for illustration. Suppose, out of 1,000 people in the unvaccinated group, 10 developed COVID-19. This gives us a disease risk of 1% in the untreated group. Now, in the vaccinated group, suppose only 6 out of 1,000 developed the disease, giving a risk of 0.6%.

The ARR is then calculated by subtracting the risk in the

vaccinated group (0.6%) from the risk in the unvaccinated group (1%). This gives us an ARR of 0.4%, meaning the vaccine reduces an individual's overall risk of disease by 0.4%.

In Pfizer's actual trial, the ARR worked out to be 0.84%, a figure vastly different from the 95% RRR. This means that for an individual, the vaccine reduces their overall risk of developing COVID-19 by less than one percent.

These numbers can be surprising, especially when juxtaposed with the 95% figure we've heard so much about. However, they are not necessarily cause for alarm or a sign that the vaccine is ineffective. They simply paint a more nuanced picture of what vaccine efficacy means and show how different measures can lead to different interpretations.

Ultimately, the 0.84% ARR does not make for a catchy headline or a reassuring soundbite. It is, nonetheless, a crucial part of understanding the full impact and limitations of Pfizer's COVID-19 vaccine. As we navigate through the complexities of this pandemic and the interventions designed to mitigate it, appreciating the full story behind the numbers is paramount.

CHAPTER 6: THE GRAND ILLUSION

In the grand theater of public health communication, the 95% efficacy claim took center stage, dazzling the audience with a promise of potent protection. The narrative spun was that of a mighty shield, fending off the dread of COVID-19 for nearly everyone who held it. Yet, lurking in the shadows, the humble figure of 0.84% waited in silence, a humble understudy to the headline act.

What unfolded was the creation of an illusion, a grand spectacle where the Relative Risk Reduction was dressed as the champion of overall protection. This misconception wasn't born out of malicious intent or dubious data. Rather, it emerged from a time-honored tradition in scientific communication, where RRR often takes the limelight.

The critical issue, however, lies in the absence of context and clarity. The public, thirsty for relief and reassurance, was offered a glass brimming with 95% efficacy. But this drink was heady with confusion, as the fine print of its true meaning blurred into obscurity. Without understanding the distinction between RRR and ARR, the audience was left to marvel at the illusion of an almost invincible defense.

In this spectacle, one can discern an insidious form of data manipulation—not through the alteration of figures but their presentation. The singular focus on RRR, coupled with the lack of clear explanations, served to create a specific narrative. It was a narrative that amplified public optimism, boosted vaccine uptake, and perhaps inadvertently, instilled a false sense of individual invulnerability.

In essence, the presentation of Pfizer's vaccine efficacy illustrates a larger issue in scientific communication: the oversimplification of complex data for mass consumption, leading to misconceptions and potentially misguided decisions.

As we pull back the curtain on this grand illusion, it is not to undermine the importance or credibility of Pfizer's vaccine, but to emphasize the need for transparency, accuracy, and context in public health communication. It is a call for scientific truths to be delivered complete, not as fragments that, when isolated, can paint a misleading picture. For it is only with the full, unobscured view can we make informed decisions and realistic expectations, the ultimate defense in our battle against COVID-19.

CHAPTER 7: THE FALLOUT

The fallout from the revelation of the 0.84% ARR was like a stone dropped into a still pond, rippling through the scientific community and the general public alike. Among those who understood the distinction between RRR and ARR, there was a collective gasp of surprise. Many felt deceived, as if the wool had been pulled over their eyes, even if the data had always been there, lurking in the shadows of the original trial report.

The public's reaction was a cocktail of confusion, betrayal, and skepticism. The bright beacon of hope that the 95% efficacy claim represented suddenly seemed less radiant, tarnished by the revelation of its true meaning. For some, trust in public health institutions wavered, fueling vaccine hesitancy and conspiracy theories. Yet, for others, it ignited a newfound desire for understanding, an urgency to peek behind the curtain of scientific data and public health communications.

In the scientific community, the discourse was, predictably, more nuanced. Some experts argued that the use of RRR is standard in such trials and studies, defending its presentation as the primary efficacy measure. Others, however, criticized the lack of clarity and transparency, calling for more accessible and complete public communication of such critical data.

This dichotomy of responses illuminated the ethical implications of such representational choices in healthcare. At the heart of it, the question arose: how much simplification is too much, especially when the stakes are high and global? This Pandora's Box of ethical queries challenged the healthcare community to introspect, to re-evaluate the balance between readability and accuracy in health communication.

As the dust settled on the initial shock, one thing became increasingly clear: transparency in public health communication is not an option, but a necessity. When data is presented in a misleading or oversimplified manner, it creates a domino effect that shakes the very foundations of public trust and comprehension. Thus, the fallout from the Pfizer efficacy illusion was not just about a statistical misunderstanding but a larger lesson in health communication ethics, accountability, and public trust.

CHAPTER 8: THE WAY FORWARD

As we turn the final pages of this exploration into Pfizer's trial report, it's crucial that we don't just close the book and return to the status quo. The discrepancies we've unraveled, the incongruity between Relative and Absolute Risk Reduction, should serve as a wake-up call for all of us. The journey does not end here; instead, it prompts us towards a new direction – the way forward.

Healthcare decisions, especially in the midst of a global pandemic, carry immense weight. As individuals, we bear the responsibility of ensuring that our choices are well-informed, based not on a single headline or a compelling statistic, but a comprehensive understanding of the facts. We need to question, probe, and demand clarity when faced with ambiguous or misleading data.

However, the onus isn't solely on the public. The healthcare sector, too, must rise to the occasion. Pharmaceutical companies, researchers, and regulatory authorities should uphold stringent standards of transparency. The presentation of clinical trial data should be clear, accurate, and devoid of any attempts to paint a skewed narrative. Every piece of data, no matter how insignificant it may appear, should be disclosed and explained. After all, as we've seen, sometimes it's the 0.84% truths that hold the most significance.

Reform, though challenging, is not impossible. Changes can be initiated at multiple levels. Regulatory bodies can implement stricter guidelines for data reporting. Researchers can commit to ethical standards that prioritize patient understanding over corporate interests. As for the public, we can wield our collective power to demand honesty and accountability.

Our journey through the labyrinth of Pfizer's COVID-19 vaccine efficacy rate has revealed much. It has shown us the power of numbers, the ease with which they can create illusions, and the dire need for transparency. As we move forward, let's not forget these lessons. Instead, let's use them as a beacon, guiding us towards a future where health decisions are made not in the shadow of manipulated data, but in the light of transparent, comprehensive truth.

EPILOGUE: LESSONS LEARNED

As we bring this exploration of Pfizer's COVID-19 vaccine efficacy to a close, it's critical to reflect on the lessons this saga has taught us. It was an episode that transcended the mere numbers involved, metamorphosing into an emblematic case study in scientific communication and public trust.

This journey has taught us the necessity for precise, transparent scientific communication. A single choice of words, a single presentation of data can dramatically shift the public's perception and understanding. The lesson here is simple: transparency isn't an optional add-on; it's an integral part of scientific discourse. Every term, every statistic we use, matters. The Relative versus Absolute Risk Reduction debate is a potent reminder of this reality.

We've also learned the importance of critical thinking, of not accepting everything at face value. The necessity of delving beneath the surface, of seeking out the Absolute Risk Reductions hidden behind the more enticing Relative ones. In an era teeming with information and misinformation alike, this critical approach isn't merely useful; it's essential.

Perhaps the most poignant lesson, however, revolves around trust. Public trust in science and healthcare is a fragile, invaluable asset. Once lost, it's arduously hard to regain. Misleading narratives, such as the one we've dissected, can erode this trust and fuel skepticism. Thus, every effort must be made to ensure that this trust isn't compromised.

In conclusion, the "Pfizer's Efficacy Illusion: The 0.84% Truth" saga offers us vital lessons on scientific communication, critical thinking, and trust. As we move forward, let's strive to remember these lessons. Let's ensure that they inform our approach to healthcare, shaping a future where scientific discourse is not only transparent and accurate but also respects and upholds the public's trust. In the end, it's not just about getting the numbers right; it's about doing right by the people those numbers serve.

ABOUT THE AUTHOR

Alex Exum

Alex Exum is a critical thinker, independent researcher, and outspoken advocate for truth and transparency in healthcare. Known for his thought-provoking discourse and relentless pursuit of knowledge, Alex's unique perspective has 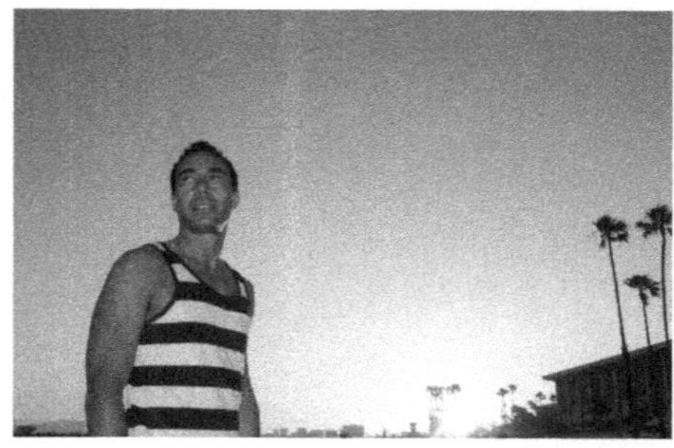 illuminated numerous controversies within the medical field. With a keen eye for detail and an unwavering commitment to unmasking misleading narratives, he has become a leading voice in the quest for unbiased healthcare information.

With his latest work, "Pfizer's Efficacy Illusion: The 0.84% Truth," Alex takes readers on a riveting journey through the intricate details of Pfizer's original COVID-19 vaccine trial report. Tackling complex concepts with an approachable style, Alex aims to empower the average person to understand and question the information presented to them.

Alex's work is driven by a simple but profound belief: knowledge should not be exclusive. It should be accessible, understandable, and accurate. By challenging existing narratives and provoking critical thinking, Alex hopes to bring about a new era of transparency and integrity in healthcare communication.

When he isn't unraveling medical controversies, Alex can be found hosting engaging discussions on his popular talk show, navigating a range of subjects with a unique blend of humor, wit, and insightful commentary. Alex Exum continues to be a beacon of truth, challenging the status quo, and fostering a community where free thought isn't just welcomed, but celebrated.

https://www.alexexum.com/